A Journey into Understanding Healthy Eating Habits

Discover the Joy of Nutrient-Rich Foods and Sustainable Lifestyle Choices

Brenda F. Dozier

Table of Contents

Introduction

There is a cornerstone of well-being that is frequently overlooked in the maze of modern living, amidst the clamor of information and the hustle and bustle of daily existence. The cornerstone is the relevance of maintaining appropriate eating habits. Dear reader, I would like to extend a warm welcome to you as you engage in fascinating learning and discovery into the worlds of nutrition and sustenance. The trip that we are on is not only about the food that we consume; rather, it is a study into how we nourish our bodies, minds, and spirits. As we set out on this journey together, let us begin by removing the layers of misunderstanding and delving into the core of what it means to accept good eating habits as the basis for a life that is rich in meaning.

Welcome to your journey

I would like to extend a warm welcome to you as you embark on a journey that goes beyond every day and challenges your preconceived views about nutrition. You are urged to become both the explorer and the architect of your own well-being as you begin on this journey, which is an expedition into the undiscovered frontiers of your own relationship with food. I would like to extend a hand of fellowship and support to you as we embark on this trip together. This path is about self-discovery just as much as it is about grasping the complexities of healthy eating habits.

It is up to you to succeed in this path, and you should be guided by your curiosity, your intuition, and your desire to learn. This presents a chance for you to take charge of your health and wellness, equipping yourself with the knowledge and resources necessary to make well-informed decisions that are in line with your individual preferences and requirements. So, welcome, dear traveler, to a journey of self-exploration, growth, and transformation—a trip that begins with a single step towards a better, happier you.

Understanding the Importance of Healthy Eating Habits

At the heart of our research lies a profound truth—a fact that transcends trends and fads, and speaks to the core of our existence: the importance of healthy eating habits. It's a reality that echoes in every cell of our body, impacting our physical health, emotional well-being, and total vitality. Understanding its relevance is not only an intellectual exercise; it's a crucial component of recovering our power and agency in designing our lives.

Healthy eating habits serve as the cornerstone of a vigorous, full existence. They are the gasoline that powers our bodies, delivering the critical elements needed for optimal performance and vigor. Each bite we take is an opportunity to nourish ourselves from the inside out, restore our cells, and assist our body's natural healing mechanisms. Moreover, healthy eating habits lay the foundation for long-term health and wellness, minimizing the risk of chronic diseases and boosting our overall quality of life.

Beyond the physical realm, good eating habits play a significant role in supporting our mental and emotional well-being. The foods we consume immediately impact our emotions, energy levels, and cognitive function, influencing our capacity to navigate life's problems with resilience and clarity. By embracing good eating habits, we nurture not just our bodies but also our minds, generating a sense of balance, stability, and emotional vibrancy.

In our fast-paced, modern society, the importance of healthy eating habits cannot be stressed. Amidst the rush and bustle of daily life, it's easy to value convenience above

sustenance, opting for processed foods and quick fixes that offer short satisfaction but fail to nourish us at a deeper level. However, true feeding goes beyond mere sustenance; it's about honoring our bodies, respecting the natural rhythms of our physiology, and building a thoughtful relationship with food.

As we continue on this path of understanding the importance of healthy eating habits, let us approach it with an open heart and a curious mind. Let us welcome the opportunity to review our connection with food, challenge old habits and ideas, and cultivate a greater knowledge of the enormous impact that our dietary choices have on our lives. Together, let us begin on this trip of self-discovery and empowerment, guided by the wisdom of our bodies and the promise of a healthier, more vibrant future.

Chapter 1

The Science of Nutrition

Nutrition, frequently referred to as the fundamental principle of health, is a broad field that involves the study of how food nourishes and sustains the human body. At its core, nutrition digs into the various mechanisms by which nutrients are absorbed, processed, and utilized by the body to support important functions and promote general well-being. Understanding the science of nutrition is not only an academic pursuit but a gateway to educated decision-making regarding dietary choices and their impact on health outcomes.

Exploring Macronutrients and Micronutrients

At the cornerstone of nutrition lie two unique groups of nutrients—macronutrients and micronutrients. Macronutrients, as the name suggests, are the nutrients that our bodies require in huge quantities to support life. These include carbs, proteins, and lipids, each performing a specific role in feeding our bodies and supporting important activities.

Carbohydrates, sometimes maligned in the area of popular diets, serve as the major source of energy for our bodies. They are found in several foods, ranging from fruits and vegetables to grains and legumes. When consumed, carbohydrates are broken down into glucose—a type of sugar that acts as the body's main energy source. While some advocate for low-carbohydrate diets, it's crucial to realize the role of carbs in maintaining sustained energy levels and supporting overall metabolic health.

Proteins, on the other hand, are the building elements of life. They play a key function in the growth, repair, and maintenance of our body tissues, including muscles, organs, and skin. Proteins are composed of amino acids, some of which are essential, meaning they must be received from our diet as our bodies cannot create them. Animal sources such as meat, fish, and dairy products are high in complete proteins, including all required amino acids, while plant-based sources like legumes, nuts, and seeds can supply a broad array of amino acids when ingested in combination.

Fats, often misunderstood and misrepresented, are necessary for various body functions, including hormone production, cell membrane integrity, and nutrient absorption. While they are more calorie-dense than carbs and proteins, fats provide a concentrated source of energy and contribute to feelings of satiety when ingested in moderation. It's vital to distinguish between healthy fats, such as those found in avocados, nuts, seeds, and fatty fish, and bad fats, such as trans fats and excessive saturated fats, which can lead to inflammation and cardiovascular disease risk.

In addition to macronutrients, our systems rely on a multitude of micronutrients—vitamins and minerals that are required in lesser quantities but are no less necessary for overall health. Micronutrients serve as cofactors and catalysts in innumerable metabolic events, regulating everything from immune function to bone health to energy metabolism.

Vitamins are chemical molecules that perform crucial functions in many physiological processes. For example, vitamin C is important for collagen synthesis, wound healing, and immunological function, while vitamin D regulates calcium intake and supports bone health. Minerals, on the other hand, are inorganic components that are necessary for several body functions. Minerals such as calcium, magnesium, and phosphorus are necessary for bone health, while others like iron, zinc, and selenium play roles in energy production, immunological function, and antioxidant defense.

Understanding Digestion and Absorption

Once we swallow food, it goes on a spectacular journey through our digestive system—a process regulated by a complicated interplay of organs, enzymes, and hormones. Digestion occurs in the mouth when enzymes in saliva begin to break down carbs into smaller molecules. From there, the food goes down the esophagus and into the stomach, where gastric acids further break down proteins and lipids.

As food exits the stomach and enters the small intestine, it encounters a milieu of digestive enzymes and bile produced by the liver and stored in the gallbladder. These enzymes work hard to break down macronutrients into their constituent parts—carbohydrates into sugars, proteins into amino acids, and fats into fatty acids and glycerol.

Once broken down, these nutrients are absorbed through the walls of the small intestine and into the bloodstream, where they are delivered to cells throughout the body for usage as energy or building blocks for tissue repair and growth. The absorption of nutrients is a carefully regulated process, with specific transport systems ensuring that only the necessary molecules are absorbed while others are expelled as waste.

Micronutrients, such as vitamins and minerals, follow a similar path but typically require particular transporters and binding proteins to enhance their absorption. For example, fat-soluble vitamins (vitamins A, D, E, and K) are absorbed together with dietary lipids and are subsequently carried through the lymphatic system before entering the bloodstream. In contrast, water-soluble vitamins (such as B vitamins and vitamin C) are absorbed directly into the bloodstream and are commonly eliminated in the urine if ingested in excess.

The voyage of digestion and absorption is a perfectly orchestrated symphony—a monument to the remarkable complexity and efficiency of the human body. Yet, despite its complexity, this mechanism is not perfect, and different circumstances can alter nutrient absorption. Certain medical diseases, such as celiac disease or inflammatory bowel disease, can limit nutrient absorption, while drugs or dietary variables may interfere with the absorption of specific nutrients.

The science of nutrition offers a fascinating view into the inner workings of our bodies and the tremendous impact of dietary choices on our health and well-being. By knowing the roles of macronutrients and micronutrients and the subtleties of digestion and absorption, we obtain vital insights for adjusting our meals for optimal health. Through informed decisions and attentive eating practices, we may harness the power of nutrition to fuel our bodies, feed our brains, and develop a thriving life.

Chapter 2

Nutrient-Rich Foods

In the enormous terrain of dietary choices, one element holds firm: the importance of nutrient-rich foods in fostering health and vitality. Nutrient-rich foods are those that contain a high concentration of key vitamins, minerals, and other vital nutrients relative to their caloric content. They form the foundation of a balanced diet, giving a wealth of health advantages that reach far beyond simply nutrition. In this research, we dig into the area of nutrient-rich foods, exploring the essential nutrients that minerals and vitamins contain and contrasting them with the hazards of processed foods.

Nutrient-rich foods comprise a varied array of whole, minimally processed foods that are packed with critical elements necessary for optimal health. These foods are generally rich in vitamins, minerals, antioxidants, fiber, and phytonutrients, all of which play vital roles in supporting various biological functions and boosting overall well-being. From bright fruits and vegetables to nourishing whole grains and lean meats, nutrient-rich foods offer a symphony of aromas and textures that nourish both the body and the soul.

Essential Vitamins and Minerals

Among the key components of nutrient-rich foods are vitamins and minerals—micronutrients that are needed for several physiological processes within the body. Vitamins are chemical substances that act as coenzymes, enabling numerous metabolic activities and maintaining overall health. They are grouped into two categories: water-soluble vitamins (such as B vitamins and vitamin C) and fat-soluble vitamins (containing vitamins A, D, E, and K).

Water-soluble vitamins are not retained in the body to the same amount as fat-soluble vitamins and must be supplied frequently through the food. They have crucial functions in energy metabolism, immunological function, and neuronal transmission. For example, vitamin C is needed for collagen synthesis, wound healing, and immunological function, while the B vitamins (such as thiamine, riboflavin, niacin, B6, B12, biotin, and pantothenic acid) are elaborate in energy production, DNA synthesis, and nervous system function.

In contrast, fat-soluble vitamins are stored in the body's adipose tissue and liver and are absorbed together with dietary lipids. These vitamins are necessary for different body activities, including eyesight (vitamin A), bone health (vitamin D), antioxidant defense (vitamin E), and blood coagulation (vitamin K). While fat-soluble vitamins are stored in the body, it's vital to eat them periodically to maintain optimum levels and support good health.

Minerals, on the other hand, are inorganic elements that serve as cofactors for enzyme reactions, control fluid balance, and contribute to bone health, neuron function, and muscle contraction. They are categorized into two categories: major minerals (such as calcium, magnesium, phosphorus, potassium, sodium, and chloride) and trace minerals (including iron, zinc, copper, selenium, iodine, manganese, and chromium).

Major minerals are required in bigger quantities and serve essential roles in numerous physiological processes. For example, calcium is needed for bone health, muscle function, and nerve transmission, while potassium is necessary for fluid balance, muscle contraction, and blood pressure regulation. Trace minerals, although necessary in lower amounts, are as vital for health and well-being. For instance, iron is needed for oxygen transport, energy metabolism, and immunological function, whereas zinc is involved in DNA synthesis, wound healing, and immune response.

Whole Foods vs. Processed Foods

In contradiction to nutrient-rich whole meals, processed foods are those that have undergone major adjustments during manufacture, typically resulting in a loss of important nutrients and the inclusion of undesirable substances such as refined sugars, bad fats, sodium, and artificial additives. Processed foods comprise a wide range of products, including sugary snacks, refined grains, packaged meals, and fast food items.

Whole foods, on the other hand, are minimally processed or unprocessed foods that keep their inherent nutrient content and offer several health benefits. These include fruits, vegetables, whole grains, legumes, nuts, seeds, lean proteins, and healthy fats. Whole foods are rich in critical nutrients, dietary fiber, and phytonutrients, all of which contribute to general health and well-being.

One of the key differences between whole foods and processed foods resides in their nutrient content. Whole foods are naturally rich in important vitamins, minerals, antioxidants, and other useful substances, but processed meals often lack these elements due to refining, heating, and other manufacturing procedures. For example, whole grains have bran, germ, and endosperm, which give fiber, vitamins, minerals, and phytonutrients, whereas refined grains are stripped of these nutrients during processing.

Moreover, processed meals often contain added sugars, harmful fats, sodium, and artificial additives, which can lead to different health concerns such as obesity, heart disease, diabetes, and inflammation. The high sugar content of many processed meals can contribute to rapid rises and crashes in blood sugar levels, encouraging cravings, hunger, and weight gain. Similarly, the excessive intake of harmful fats, such as trans fats and saturated fats, might increase the risk of heart disease and other chronic illnesses.

In contrast, whole foods provide a balanced array of nutrients that support general health and well-being. They are naturally lacking in added sugars, harmful fats, and artificial additives, making them a healthier choice for maintaining maximum health. Incorporating a variety of whole foods into your diet will help ensure proper intake of important vitamins, minerals, antioxidants, and other beneficial substances, while minimizing the consumption of processed foods can help lessen the risk of chronic diseases and increase longevity.

Nutrient-rich foods provide the cornerstone of a nutritious diet, supplying necessary vitamins, minerals, antioxidants, and other beneficial components that support general health and well-being. By focusing on whole, minimally processed foods and including a variety of fruits, vegetables, whole grains, legumes, nuts, seeds, lean proteins, and healthy fats in your diet, you may optimize your nutrient intake and promote maximum health. Making informed decisions about the foods you consume and choosing nutrient-rich selections can help you attain and maintain a healthy weight, boost immunological function, minimize the risk of chronic diseases, and enhance overall vitality and well-being.

Chapter 3

Building a Balanced Plate

Building a balanced plate is a core part of healthy eating, one that involves not only the quantity but also the quality and diversity of foods we consume. It is an art and a science, requiring attention, understanding, and intentionality to produce meals that nourish our bodies and enhance our general well-being. In this inquiry, we look into the concepts of building a balanced plate, the necessity of portion control and food groupings, and the transforming effect of colorful eating.

At the heart of Building a balanced plate is the concept of balance itself—a harmonious combination of macronutrients, micronutrients, and other vital components that promote good health. A balanced plate is not only about loading up on an array of foods; it is about carefully picking a variety of nutrient-dense foods that provide a wide range of important nutrients and support overall health and well-being.

A balanced meal often consists of four primary components: vegetables, fruits, lean proteins, and whole grains or starchy vegetables. These components interact synergistically to deliver a varied array of nutrients, including vitamins, minerals, antioxidants, fiber, and phytonutrients, all of which play vital roles in supporting various biological functions and improving overall health.

Vegetables constitute the cornerstone of a balanced plate, supplying critical vitamins, minerals, fiber, and antioxidants with minimum calories and fat. They are rich in vitamins A, C, and K, as well as folate, potassium, and fiber, all of which help with immune function, bone health, heart health, and digestive health. Aim to fill half of your plate with colorful, non-starchy veggies such as leafy greens, broccoli, bell peppers, carrots, and tomatoes to maximize your nutritional intake and increase satiety.

Fruits are another crucial component of a balanced plate, delivering a sweet and refreshing accompaniment to meals and snacks. They are rich in vitamins, minerals, antioxidants, and fiber, all of which contribute to general health and well-being. Fruits are particularly rich in vitamin C, potassium, and fiber, which boost immune function, heart health, and digestive health. Aim to incorporate a variety of colorful fruits such as berries, oranges, apples, bananas, and grapes in your diet to maximize your vitamin intake and healthfully fulfill your sweet tooth.

Lean proteins are essential for creating and repairing tissues, supporting muscular growth and maintenance, and promoting satiety and weight management. They are rich in important amino acids, which are the building blocks of protein and are also a good source of vitamins and minerals such as iron, zinc, and B vitamins. Aim to include a variety of lean proteins such as poultry, fish, tofu, beans, lentils, and low-fat dairy products in your diet to meet your protein demands and support general health and well-being.

Whole grains and starchy vegetables provide a great source of complex carbs, fiber, vitamins, and minerals that support energy production, digestive health, and general well-being. They are also a good source of phytonutrients, which have been demonstrated to have many health advantages, including reducing the risk of chronic diseases like as heart disease, diabetes, and cancer. Aim to incorporate a range of whole grains such as brown rice, quinoa, oats, and barley, as well as starchy vegetables such as sweet potatoes, potatoes, and winter squash, in your diet to maximize your nutritional intake and promote fullness and satisfaction.

In addition to these four primary components, a balanced plate also includes healthy fats and beverages. Healthy fats, such as those found in nuts, seeds, avocados, and olive oil, contain vital fatty acids, vitamins, and antioxidants that support brain function, heart health, and overall well-being. Aim to include a range of healthy fats in your diet to support general health and well-being. Beverages such as water, herbal tea, and unsweetened beverages are necessary for hydration and overall health and well-being. Aim to drink lots of water throughout the day to stay hydrated and support good health and well-being.

Portion Control and Food Groups

In addition to designing a balanced plate, portion control plays a significant part in keeping a healthy weight and promoting general health and well-being. Portion control entails consuming the proper amount of food to meet your energy demands without overeating or under-eating. It is crucial to listen to your body's hunger and fullness cues and to be careful of portion sizes to support general health and well-being.

One strategy to learn portion control is to utilize visual cues and portion sizes to guide your eating decisions. For example, strive to fill half of your plate with non-starchy veggies, one quarter with lean protein, and one-quarter with whole grains or starchy vegetables. This visual approach can help you build a balanced plate and limit portion sizes without tracking calories or measuring servings.

Another strategy to practice portion control is to pay attention to serving sizes and portion sizes when eating out or making meals at home. Many restaurants and packaged foods offer excessive servings that might lead to overeating and weight gain. It is crucial to be attentive to serving sizes and portion sizes and to pick smaller quantities when possible to improve general health and well-being.

In addition to portion control, food categories play a significant role in establishing a balanced plate and supporting general health and well-being. Food groups are categories of foods that exhibit similar nutritional features and are grouped based on their nutrient content and significance in the diet. The five main food groups include fruits, vegetables, grains, protein foods, and dairy or dairy alternatives.

Fruits and vegetables are key sources of essential vitamins, minerals, antioxidants, and fiber that support general health and well-being. They are rich in critical nutrients such as vitamin C, potassium, and fiber, which support immune function, heart health, and digestive health. Aim to incorporate a variety of colorful fruits and vegetables in your diet to maximize your nutritional intake and enhance overall health and well-being.

Grains are another key food type that provides a great source of complex carbs, fiber, vitamins, and minerals that support general health and well-being. Whole grains such as brown rice, quinoa, oats, and barley are particularly rich in fiber, vitamins, and minerals and are connected with a lower risk of chronic diseases such as heart disease, diabetes, and cancer. Aim to include a variety of whole grains in your diet to maximize your nutrient intake and enhance overall health and well-being.

Protein meals are needed for creating and repairing tissues, supporting muscular growth and maintenance, and promoting satiety and weight management. They are rich in important amino acids, which are the building blocks of protein and are also a good source of vitamins and minerals such as iron, zinc, and B vitamins. Aim to include a variety of lean proteins such as poultry, fish, tofu, beans, lentils, and low-fat dairy products in your diet to meet your protein demands and support general health and well-being.

Dairy or dairy alternatives are another vital food group that provides a rich source of essential nutrients such as calcium, vitamin D, and protein that promote bone health, muscle function, and general health and well-being. Dairy products such as milk, yogurt, and cheese are rich in calcium and vitamin D, which are vital for bone health and overall health and well-being. If you are lactose intolerant or prefer not to consume dairy products, there are numerous dairy replacements available, such as soy milk, almond milk, and oat milk, that provide equivalent nutrients and can be incorporated into a balanced diet.

In addition to these five primary food groups, healthy fats such as those found in nuts, seeds, avocados, and olive oil, are a crucial part of a balanced diet. These fats contain vital fatty acids, vitamins, and antioxidants that support brain function, heart health, and overall well-being. While fats are calorie-dense, they play a critical role in satiety and should be incorporated in moderation as part of a balanced meal.

It's necessary to emphasize that portion control and dietary groupings are not about harsh restrictions or hardship. Instead, they serve as suggestions to help you make informed decisions and construct balanced meals that support your overall health and well-being. By paying attention to portion sizes and including a range of nutrient-rich foods from different food categories in your diet, you may maximize your nutrient intake and promote optimal health.

The Power of Colorful Eating

In the field of nutrition, the expression "eat the rainbow" is widely used to indicate the importance of adding a range of colored fruits and vegetables into your diet. This approach, known as a colorful diet, highlights the health advantages of consuming a varied assortment of fruits and vegetables, each offering a distinct combination of vitamins, minerals, antioxidants, and phytonutrients.

Colorful eating is not only about aesthetics; it's about harnessing the power of nature's palette to enhance health and energy. Different colors in fruits and vegetables are typically indicative of the presence of specific nutrients and antioxidants, each with its own set of health advantages. For example, orange and yellow fruits and vegetables such as carrots, sweet potatoes, and oranges are rich in beta-carotene, which supports eye health and immunological function.

Similarly, red fruits and vegetables such as tomatoes, strawberries, and red bell peppers are rich in lycopene and anthocyanins, which have been associated with a lower risk of chronic diseases such as heart disease and cancer. Green vegetables such as spinach, kale, and broccoli are rich in chlorophyll, fiber, vitamins, and minerals that support bone health, digestive health, and general well-being.

By including a variety of colored fruits and vegetables in your diet, you may ensure a diverse intake of key nutrients and antioxidants that support general health and well-being. Aim to include a range of colors in your meals and snacks each day to maximize your nutritional intake and support optimal health.

In addition to fruits and vegetables, colorful eating also extends to other dietary groups, including grains, protein foods, and healthy fats. Whole grains such as quinoa, brown rice, and oats come in a range of colors, each giving a unique combination of nutrients and fiber that support digestive health and general well-being.

Protein foods such as beans, lentils, tofu, and lean meats also come in a range of hues, each giving a unique combination of amino acids, vitamins, and minerals that support muscle growth and repair, immunological function, and general health and well-being. Healthy fats such as those found in nuts, seeds, avocados, and olive oil contain important fatty acids, vitamins, and antioxidants that support brain function, heart health, and overall well-being.

Building a balanced plate, practicing portion control, and embracing the power of colorful food are vital components of a healthy diet and lifestyle. By including a range of nutrient-rich foods from different food categories in your diet and paying attention to portion sizes, you may maximize your nutrient intake and promote maximum health and well-being. Remember, healthy eating is not about limitation or deprivation; it's about providing your body with the nutrition it needs to thrive and embracing the power of food as medicine.

Chapter 4

Mindful Eating Techniques

Mindful eating practices have gained favor in recent years as a holistic approach to nourishing the body and creating a healthy relationship with food. Rooted in the practice of mindfulness—a state of non-judgmental awareness of the present moment—mindful eating encourages individuals to bring focused attention to their eating experiences, establishing a deeper connection with their bodies and the food they consume. In this study, we look into the principles of mindful eating, the practice of mindful awareness, and the necessity of listening to your body's hunger cues.

Mindful eating is neither a diet nor a set of stringent restrictions but rather a mentality and a collection of activities aimed to encourage increased awareness and appreciation of the eating experience. It involves paying full attention to the sensory experience of eating—savoring the flavors, textures, and scents of food, as well as noticing hunger and fullness cues, and fostering a non-judgmental attitude towards food and eating habits.

One of the core concepts of mindful eating is eating deliberately and savoring each bite. Rather than rushing through meals or mindlessly ingesting food, mindful eaters take the time to chew deeply, completely enjoy the taste and texture of each bite, and pay attention to how the food makes them feel. By slowing down and savoring each bite, individuals can build a better appreciation for the food they consume and become more attentive to their body's hunger and fullness signals.

Another crucial part of mindful eating is paying attention to hunger and fullness cues. This entails tuning into the body's innate signals of hunger and satiety eating only when hungry and stopping when satisfied. Mindful eaters seek to eat when their body signals hunger and to finish eating when they feel pleasantly full, rather than relying on extrinsic cues such as portion sizes or mealtimes. By listening to their body's natural hunger and fullness cues, individuals can create a healthier relationship with food and prevent overeating or undereating.

Additionally, mindful eating involves being attentive to the emotional and psychological components of eating. This includes recognizing and acknowledging emotional triggers for eating, such as stress, boredom, or melancholy, and learning to respond to these triggers in non-food-related ways. Mindful eaters seek to eat for physical hunger rather than emotional hunger and to approach food with a sense of inquiry, openness, and self-compassion.

Practicing mindfulness during meals can also involve creating a tranquil and mindful eating environment. This may include setting the table with care, eliminating distractions such as screens or technological gadgets, and eating in a peaceful and relaxed atmosphere. By creating a mindful eating environment, individuals can enhance their awareness of the eating experience and build a stronger feeling of connection with their food and their bodies.

The Practice of Mindful Awareness

Mindful awareness is a core part of mindful eating, comprising the practice of non-judgmental awareness of the current moment. Mindful awareness entails bringing concentrated attention to the sensory experience of eating, including the taste, texture, smell, and look of food, as well as the bodily feelings and emotions that develop during the eating process.

One of the basic concepts of mindful awareness is non-judgmental observation. This includes monitoring the present moment without attaching judgment or criticism to the experience. For example, rather than categorizing things as "good" or "bad" or blaming oneself for eating certain foods, individuals practice just observing their thoughts, feelings, and experiences without judgment.

Another facet of conscious awareness is acceptance and compassion. This means embracing the current moment as it is, without trying to modify or reject it, and growing self-compassion and goodwill towards oneself. For example, if individuals see themselves evaluating their eating habits or feeling guilty about their food choices, they practice reacting with self-compassion and kindness, realizing that everyone makes mistakes and that it's important to learn and grow from them.

Practicing mindful awareness during meals also involves bringing focused attention to the bodily sensations and emotions that arise when eating. This includes noting feelings such as hunger, fullness, pleasure, and pain, as well as emotions such as joy, sadness, or tension. By bringing awareness to these feelings and emotions, individuals can develop a stronger knowledge of their eating habits and patterns and make more conscious choices regarding food and eating.

In addition to practicing mindful awareness at meals, individuals can also cultivate mindfulness in other areas of their lives to promote their overall well-being. This may include practicing mindfulness meditation, yoga, or other mindfulness-based activities, as well as bringing awareness into regular activities such as walking, cooking, or spending time in nature. By practicing mindfulness in all parts of life, individuals can acquire a better feeling of presence, calm, and well-being.

Listening to Your Body's Hunger Cues

Listening to your body's hunger cues is a key component of mindful eating, as it includes tuning into the body's natural signals of hunger and fullness and responding to them correctly. Hunger signals are the body's way of signaling that it needs sustenance, whereas fullness cues suggest that the body has had enough food and is satiated.

One of the basic aspects of responding to your body's hunger cues is eating when hungry and stopping when content. This involves tuning into the bodily symptoms of hunger, such as stomach growling, lightheadedness, or low energy, and responding to these cues by eating a balanced meal or snack. Similarly, individuals practice paying attention to the physical sensations of fullness, such as feeling comfortably filled or no longer feeling hungry, and stopping eating when these signs come.

Added component of responding to your body's hunger cues is distinguishing between physical hunger and other types of hunger, such as emotional hunger or boredom. Physical hunger is defined by physical feelings such as stomach growling, lightheadedness, or poor energy, while emotional hunger is generally accompanied by desires for certain foods, eating out of boredom or stress, or feeling guilty or ashamed about eating. By learning to recognize the distinction between physical hunger and other types of hunger, individuals can make more conscientious choices regarding food and eating.

Practicing mindfulness during meals can also help individuals tune into their body's hunger cues and respond to them correctly. By bringing concentrated attention to the sensory experience of eating and observing physical sensations such as hunger and fullness, individuals can acquire a higher understanding of their body's requirements and make more conscious choices regarding food and eating. Additionally, exercising mindfulness can help individuals create a higher sense of contentment and enjoyment from their meals, leading to a more balanced and gratifying eating experience.

Mindful eating practices, the practice of mindful awareness, and listening to your body's hunger cues are vital components of a healthy relationship with food and eating. By bringing focused attention to the sensory experience of eating, practicing mindfulness in all aspects of life, and tuning into the body's natural signals of hunger and fullness, individuals can create a deeper sense of presence, calm, and well-being surrounding food and eating.

Chapter 5

Emotional Eating and Food Relationships

Emotional eating and food relationships are intimately connected components of human behavior that can greatly affect our overall well-being and relationship with food. The term "emotional eating" refers to the inclination to utilize food as a coping method for managing emotions such as stress, melancholy, boredom, or loneliness. This behavior normally involves consuming food in response to emotional stimuli rather than physical hunger indicators, leading to overeating or binge eating. In contrast, our food relationship involves the complex interplay of attitudes, beliefs, and actions surrounding food and eating, including our judgments of food, body image, and self-worth. In this inquiry, we look into the issue of emotional eating, tactics for handling emotional triggers, and the necessity of building a healthy relationship with food.

mental eating is a complicated and diverse behavior that can have a tremendous impact on our physical health, mental well-being, and connection with food. It frequently comes from a desire to calm or repress unwanted feelings or to seek comfort and pleasure through eating. Emotional eating may be prompted by a range of emotional states, including stress, melancholy, boredom, loneliness, worry, or even happiness. Individuals may turn to food as a way to cope with painful emotions or to reward themselves for happy experiences.

Unique of the fundamental aspects of emotional eating is the tendency to consume in reaction to emotional cues rather than physical hunger indicators. This can lead to mindless eating, where individuals consume food without being completely conscious of their hunger or fullness levels. Emotional eating generally entails eating past the point of fullness or ingesting large quantities of high-calorie, comfort foods that provide brief respite but may ultimately contribute to emotions of guilt, humiliation, or physical discomfort.

Emotional eating can also be influenced by exterior variables such as social and environmental cues, including the availability of food, social pressure to eat, or the influence of advertising and media portrayals of food. For example, individuals may be more inclined to participate in emotional eating when surrounded by tempting food options or when dining in social contexts when food is abundant and readily available.

In addition to emotional eating, our food connections cover a broader set of attitudes, beliefs, and actions surrounding food and eating. This covers our thoughts about food, body image, and self-worth, as well as our eating patterns, food choices, and cultural influences. Our food connections are shaped by a multitude of circumstances, including our childhood, cultural background, social level, and personal experiences with food and eating.

A good food relationship is characterized by a balanced and intuitive approach to eating, where individuals can enjoy food without feelings of guilt or shame, and respond to their body's hunger and fullness cues mindfully and respectfully. Cultivating a good food connection involves having a positive attitude towards food and eating, encouraging self-compassion and acceptance, and adopting mindful eating techniques that encourage better awareness of the eating experience.

Strategies for Managing Emotional Triggers

Managing emotional triggers is a key element of overcoming emotional eating and building a healthy relationship with food. It entails growing awareness of emotional triggers and employing techniques to cope with them productively and healthily. While emotional triggers may differ from person to person, common triggers include stress, melancholy, boredom, loneliness, anxiety, and other negative emotions.

One helpful method for controlling emotional triggers is to identify and acknowledge the feelings behind emotional eating patterns. This involves growing awareness of the emotional states that trigger the impulse to eat and learning to recognize the signs and symptoms of emotional distress. By understanding and embracing these emotions, individuals can begin to create more adaptive coping techniques that address the underlying emotional needs without resorting to food.

Other technique for controlling emotional triggers is to build alternate coping mechanisms for handling emotions and stress. This may involve engaging in activities that bring emotional comfort and support, such as exercise, relaxation techniques, mindfulness meditation, writing, or spending time with loved ones. By discovering healthy and productive ways to cope with emotions, individuals can minimize their dependency on food as a major coping mechanism and build more adaptive coping abilities.

In addition to establishing alternate coping methods, individuals might also benefit from implementing techniques to decrease exposure to emotional triggers. This may involve creating a supportive and nurturing environment that promotes emotional well-being, such as surrounding oneself with supportive friends and family members, practicing stress management techniques, and setting boundaries with situations or individuals that contribute to emotional distress.

Mindful eating can also be a great technique for regulating emotional triggers and maintaining a balanced relationship with food. By bringing focused attention to the eating experience and building greater awareness of hunger and fullness cues, individuals can develop a more intuitive approach to eating that is less influenced by emotional impulses. Mindful eating encourages individuals to eat with awareness and intention, relishing the flavors and textures of food and paying attention to how food makes them feel physically and emotionally.

Cultivating a Healthy Relationship with Food

Cultivating a healthy relationship with food is an ongoing process that includes self-awareness, self-compassion, and a dedication to self-care. It entails having a good attitude towards food and eating, promoting self-compassion and acceptance, and adopting mindful eating practices that encourage a better awareness of the eating experience.

One of the major elements of creating a healthy connection with food is developing a non-judgmental attitude towards food and eating habits. This means letting go of stringent dieting norms, guilt, and shame surrounding food choices, and embracing a more flexible and compassionate attitude to eating. By adopting a non-judgmental attitude towards food, individuals can lessen emotions of guilt or shame connected with eating and build a healthy connection with food and eating.

Another part of building a healthy relationship with food is fostering self-compassion and acceptance. This means treating oneself with love and empathy, especially during times of conflict or difficulty. Rather than indulging in self-criticism or negative self-talk, individuals practice reacting to themselves with empathy and self-compassion, realizing that everyone makes mistakes and that it's normal to learn and grow from them.

In addition to creating a non-judgmental attitude and encouraging self-compassion, cultivating a healthy relationship with food also requires adopting mindful eating techniques that encourage better awareness of the eating experience. Mindful eating encourages individuals to eat with awareness and intention, appreciating the flavors and textures of food, and paying attention to how food makes them feel physically and emotionally. By practicing mindful eating, individuals can build a deeper feeling of connection with their bodies and their food and make more conscientious choices about what and how they consume.

Emotional eating and food relationships are complicated components of human behavior that can greatly affect our general well-being and relationship with food. By gaining awareness of emotional triggers, employing skills for controlling emotions, and building a healthy connection with food, individuals can develop a more balanced and positive attitude to eating that supports physical and emotional well-being

Chapter 6

The Role of Physical Activity

Physical activity serves a main role in supporting overall health and well-being, involving a wide range of motions that activate the body's muscles and cardiovascular system. From regular training regimens to everyday activities such as walking or gardening, physical activity has multiple benefits for both physical and mental health. In this discussion, we look into the role of physical activity, methods of exercise in your routine, and the necessity of finding joy in movement.

Physical activity is vital for sustaining optimal health and well-being at every stage of life. It comprises any bodily activity that needs energy expenditure, ranging from low-intensity activities such as walking or stretching to more strenuous activities such as running or weightlifting. Physical activity has a critical role in enhancing physical health by boosting cardiovascular fitness, muscle strength, flexibility, and bone density. It also helps control weight, reduce the risk of chronic diseases such as heart disease, diabetes, and some types of cancer, and improve overall quality of life.

In addition to its physical benefits, physical activity also provides considerable mental health benefits. Regular exercise has been found to lessen symptoms of depression, anxiety, and stress, improve mood and cognitive performance, and promote overall psychological well-being. Physical activity stimulates the release of endorphins, chemicals in the brain that boost feelings of happiness and euphoria, resulting in what is frequently referred to as the "runner's high." Engaging in regular physical activity can also create a sense of accomplishment, raise self-esteem, and strengthen social connections by participating in group activities or sports.

Despite the multiple benefits of physical activity, many persons struggle to incorporate regular exercise into their everyday lives owing to different hurdles such as time constraints, lack of desire, or perceived difficulties. However, with proper planning and determination, it is possible to overcome these barriers and gain the pleasure of a physically active lifestyle.

Incorporating Exercise into Your Routine

Incorporating exercise into your routine needs intentionality, planning, and dedication to making physical activity a priority in your everyday life. One successful technique for incorporating exercise into your routine is to set clear, achievable goals that coincide with your interests, preferences, and fitness level. Whether your objective is to boost cardiovascular fitness, gain muscle strength, or improve flexibility, setting clear and realistic goals will help you stay motivated and focused on your fitness path.

Another technique for incorporating exercise into your routine is to make physical activity a regular component of your daily agenda. Schedule time for exercise just like you would for any other essential appointment or commitment, and treat it with the same level of priority. This may require choosing specific days and times for workouts, such as early mornings before work, during lunch breaks, or in the evenings after work. By making exercise a non-negotiable part of your daily routine, you may maintain consistency and cultivate good exercise habits over time.

Finding activities that you enjoy and that correspond with your interests and preferences is also crucial to incorporating exercise into your schedule. Whether you like solo activities such as jogging or cycling, group fitness programs such as yoga or dance, or outdoor activities such as hiking or swimming, choosing activities that you enjoy can make exercise feel less like a chore and more like a gratifying and fun experience. Experiment with numerous types of activities until you find ones that you actually enjoy and look forward to, and don't be afraid to attempt new things or go out of your comfort zone.

Incorporating exercise into your routine also includes overcoming common roadblocks and challenges that may develop along the way. This may entail finding ways to stay motivated and disciplined, being regular with your workouts, overcoming emotions of self-doubt or uncertainty, and managing time limits or competing responsibilities. By adopting strategies to address these barriers and staying focused on your goals, you can overcome hurdles and maintain a regular exercise routine that supports your overall health and well-being.

Finding Joy in Movement

Finding joy in movement is vital for having a healthy and lasting relationship with fitness. Rather than perceiving exercise as a burden or necessity, choosing activities that bring you joy and satisfaction can make physical activity feel more fun and fulfilling. Whether it's the pleasure of jogging outside, the sense of achievement from completing a hard workout, or the companionship of exercising with friends or family, finding joy in movement can enhance your overall exercise experience and drive you to continue active.

One strategy to discover joy in movement is to focus on the internal joys of exercise rather than outward outcomes such as weight loss or physical beauty. Instead of training merely for the objective of reaching a certain body shape or size, focus on how exercise makes you feel physically and mentally. Pay attention to the immediate benefits of exercise, such as greater energy, improved mood, and lower stress, and appreciate the sensations of satisfaction and well-being that come from moving your body in ways that feel good to you.

A different way to discover joy in movement is to build a sense of attention and be present throughout the exercise. Rather than going through the motions or zoning out during workouts, practice giving concentrated attention to the feelings and experiences of movement. Notice the feeling of your muscles tightening and releasing, the rhythm of your breath, and the sensations of your body moving through space. By fostering mindfulness during exercise, you can acquire a stronger appreciation for the physical and sensory sensation of movement and boost your overall exercise enjoyment.

Engaging in things that bring you joy and fulfillment can also boost your workout experience and make physical activity feel more joyful. Whether it's dancing to your favorite music, playing a sport you love, or exploring the great outdoors, choosing things that bring you joy and satisfaction can make exercise feel less like a chore and more like a satisfying and fulfilling experience. Pay attention to the things that make you feel happiest and most alive, and prioritize adding them to your fitness program regularly.

Physical activity has an important function in supporting overall health and well-being, having several advantages for both physical and mental health. By adding exercise to your routine, setting clear goals, and finding joy in moving, you may develop a positive and sustainable relationship with exercise that promotes your general health and well-being for years to come.

Chapter 7

Meal Planning and Preparation

Meal planning and preparation are important components of a healthy and balanced lifestyle, bringing several benefits such as saving time and money, decreasing stress, and fostering healthier eating habits. By making the effort to plan and prepare meals ahead of time, individuals may guarantee they have nutritious and satisfying meals easily available, making it simpler to stick to their health and wellness goals. In this exploration, we look into the importance of meal planning and preparation, offer suggestions for efficient meal prep, and provide advice on making balanced and delectable meals.

Meal planning entails determining what meals to consume in advance and gathering the necessary items and recipes to create those meals. It is a proactive strategy for controlling food choices and ensuring that individuals have access to nutritious and balanced meals throughout the week. Meal preparation, on the other hand, comprises cooking and arranging meals ahead of time to make them conveniently available for consumption.

One of the primary benefits of meal planning and preparation is that it saves time and decreases stress. By making the effort to plan meals and prepare materials ahead of time, individuals can streamline the cooking process and minimize the time spent in the kitchen during hectic weekdays. This can be especially advantageous for persons with hectic schedules or limited time for meal preparation, allowing them to enjoy healthy and home-cooked meals without the stress of last-minute meal decisions.

Meal planning and preparation also encourage healthy eating habits by giving individuals greater control over their food choices and portion levels. By planning meals, individuals can ensure they have access to nutritious and balanced meals that fit their dietary needs and preferences. This can help minimize impulsive meal choices or reliance on convenience foods that may be rich in calories, sodium, or harmful fats.

Additionally, meal planning and preparation can help individuals save money on groceries by reducing food waste and preventing wasteful expenditure on dining out or takeout meals. By choosing items thoughtfully and using them efficiently, individuals can stretch their food budget and make the most of their shopping expenditures. This can be especially advantageous for folks on a low budget or looking to save money on food bills.

Tips for Efficient Meal Prep

Efficient meal prep entails preparing and organizing meals ahead of time to streamline the cooking process and make healthy meals readily available for consumption. By following a few easy techniques and strategies, individuals can make meal prep more efficient and successful.

A possible strategy for efficient meal prep is to set aside some time each week for meal planning and preparation. This may mean setting aside a few hours on the weekend to plan meals, shopping shop, and prepare ingredients for the week ahead. By developing a consistent schedule for meal planning, individuals can make it a priority and ensure they have healthy and balanced meals easily available throughout the week.

Another suggestion for efficient meal prep is to find recipes that are simple, flexible, and easy to prepare in large numbers. Look for recipes that use common ingredients, require minimal cooking time, and can be readily tweaked to fit different preferences. Batch-cooking core foods such as grains, meats, and veggies can also save time and make it easier to prepare meals throughout the week.

In addition to batch cooking core items, prepping and portioning out ingredients ahead of time can help save time and make meal preparation more effective. Chop and wash vegetables, marinate proteins, and divide out items such as grains and legumes in advance to streamline the cooking process and make assembling meals quicker and easier.

A further choice for efficient meal planning is to invest in time-saving kitchen gear and appliances that can assist expedite the cooking process. Tools such as slow cookers, pressure cookers, and rice cookers can assist save time and make it easier to prepare meals, especially for persons with busy schedules or limited time for meal preparation.

Finally, make use of easy and time-saving meal prep tricks such as freezer meals, meal kits, and pre-packaged items to streamline the cooking process and make meal prep more efficient. Stocking up on pre-made sauces, dressings, and condiments can also save time and add flavor to meals without the need for substantial preparation.

Creating Balanced and Flavorful Meals

Creating balanced and delectable meals is crucial to enjoying healthy and fulfilling meals that support overall health and well-being. Balanced meals include a combination of macronutrients such as protein, carbs, and healthy fats, as well as a variety of vitamins, minerals, and antioxidants from fruits and vegetables.

A common approach for establishing balanced meals is to focus on including a range of nutrient-dense foods from all food groups in each meal. Aim to incorporate lean meats such as poultry, fish, tofu, or legumes, whole grains such as brown rice, quinoa, or whole wheat pasta, and lots of fruits and vegetables in a range of colors and textures. Incorporating a variety of foods from different food categories ensures that meals are nutritionally balanced and supply a wide range of critical nutrients.

Another technique for generating balanced meals is to pay attention to portion sizes and practice mindful eating. Aim to fill half of your plate with non-starchy veggies, one quarter with lean protein, and one-quarter with whole grains or starchy vegetables. This balanced plate method helps ensure that meals are portioned accurately and deliver a balanced mix of macronutrients and micronutrients.

In addition to focusing on macronutrients and portion sizes, creating delectable meals entails using herbs, spices, and seasonings to enhance taste without relying on excessive salt, sugar, or harmful fats. Experiment with different herbs and spices to add depth and complexity to your meals, and don't be afraid to get creative with flavor combinations. Incorporating fresh herbs, citrus zest, garlic, ginger, and other aromatics can boost the flavor of foods and make them more delightful to eat.

Finally, don't ignore the importance of appearance when it comes to preparing excellent meals. Taking the time to plate meals strategically and arrange components in an aesthetically pleasing manner can enhance the eating experience and make meals more fun to eat. Experiment with different plating techniques, garnishes, and serving dishes to make meals visually appealing and enticing.

Meal planning and preparation are dynamic components of a healthy and balanced lifestyle, delivering several benefits for both physical and mental health. By following these guidelines for efficient meal prep and making balanced and delectable meals, individuals may streamline the cooking process, save time and money, and enjoy nutritious and fulfilling meals that support overall health and well-being.

Chapter 8

Superfoods and Functional Foods

Superfoods and functional foods have attracted significant interest for their possible health benefits and nutritional worth. These nutrient-packed foods go beyond simple feeding, giving a range of bioactive chemicals that contribute to general well-being. In this exploration, we delve into the realm of superfoods and functional foods, analyzing their advantages and providing insights into incorporating them into a balanced and health-conscious diet.

Superfoods are a category of nutrient-dense foods that are high in vitamins, minerals, antioxidants, and other health-promoting components. While there is no formal scientific explanation for the phrase "superfood," it is widely used to describe meals that give remarkable nutritional advantages and may contribute to the prevention of certain diseases. Superfoods are generally celebrated for their high concentrations of essential nutrients relative to their calorie level.

Functional Foods Defined: Functional foods, on the other hand, are foods that go beyond basic nutrition, as they contain bioactive substances that may provide health advantages beyond plain nourishment. These foods may have specific physiological or psychological effects, such as encouraging heart health, helping digestion, or enhancing cognitive function. Functional foods are meant to optimize health and well-being and are often a component of a proactive approach to nutrition.

Exploring the Benefits of Superfoods

Rich in Antioxidants: Many superfoods are renowned for their high antioxidant content. Antioxidants help neutralize free radicals in the body, which are unstable chemicals that can cause cellular damage and contribute to different diseases, including cancer and cardiovascular disorders. Examples of antioxidant-rich superfoods include berries (blueberries, strawberries, and raspberries), dark leafy greens (kale and spinach), and nuts (walnuts and almonds).

Anti-Inflammatory Properties: Chronic inflammation is related to several health concerns, including autoimmune illnesses and certain malignancies. Superfoods such as fatty fish (salmon and mackerel), turmeric, and ginger possess anti-inflammatory benefits. Incorporating these foods into the diet may help decrease inflammation and contribute to general well-being.

Heart Health Support: Several superfoods offer benefits for cardiovascular health. Foods like oats, flaxseeds, and fatty fish include components that assist heart health by decreasing cholesterol levels, encouraging healthy blood vessels, and controlling blood pressure. Adopting a diet rich in these superfoods can be a proactive approach to sustaining cardiovascular well-being.

Brain-Boosting Nutrients: Superfoods are also recognized for their potential to boost cognitive function. Blueberries, rich in antioxidants, have been related to better memory and cognitive ability. Fatty fish contains omega-3 fatty acids and is connected with enhanced cognitive function and a lower risk of age-related cognitive decline.

Rich in Essential Nutrients: Superfoods are generally nutrient powerhouses, delivering essential vitamins and minerals required for many biological activities. Leafy greens, such as kale and spinach, are significant sources of vitamins A, C, and K, as well as minerals like iron and calcium. Including a variety of superfoods in the diet ensures a varied range of nutrients necessary for overall wellness.

Incorporating Functional Foods for Health Optimization

Probiotics for Gut Health: Functional foods typically include those containing probiotics, which are helpful bacteria that improve gut health. Yogurt, kefir, sauerkraut, and kimchi are instances of foods rich in probiotics. These microbes contribute to a healthy gut microbiome, facilitating digestion, and nutrition absorption, and even impacting mental health.

Fiber-Rich Foods: Foods high in fiber fall under the category of functional foods due to their digestive advantages. Fiber supports regular bowel motions, aids in weight management, and adds to overall gut health. Whole grains, legumes, fruits, and vegetables are good sources of nutritional fiber.

Herbs and Spices for Wellness: Functional meals also include diverse herbs and spices that give both flavor and health advantages. Turmeric contains the active component curcumin and has anti-inflammatory and antioxidant effects. Cinnamon may help manage blood sugar levels, and garlic has been related to cardiovascular health advantages.

Omega-3 Fatty Acids for Brain also Heart Health:

Functional foods high in omega-3 fatty acids aid in brain and heart health. Fatty fish like salmon and trout, flaxseeds, and chia seeds are good providers of these important fatty acids. Omega-3s serve a key role in preserving the structural integrity of cell membranes and promoting proper brain function.

Adaptogens for Stress Management: Certain functional foods are classed as adaptogens, which are considered to assist the body adapt to stress and promoting equilibrium. Examples include ashwagandha, holy basil, and rhodiola. These herbs have been used in traditional medicine to assist the body's response to stress and may aid in overall well-being.

Superfoods and functional foods have a key role in boosting health and well-being. Their varied nutritional profiles and potential health advantages make them great additions to a balanced and diverse diet. Incorporating a variety of superfoods and functional foods guarantees a wide range of necessary nutrients and bioactive substances, leading to overall health optimization. By adopting these nutrient-rich foods, individuals may adopt a proactive approach to nutrition, supporting different areas of their well-being from antioxidant protection to gut health and beyond.

Chapter 9

Hydration and Wellness

Hydration serves an essential part in sustaining overall wellness and supporting many bodily functions. Adequate hydration is crucial for good physical and mental function, as well as for improving overall health and well-being. In this inquiry, we look into the importance of adequate hydration, highlighting its advantages and proposing creative ways to stay hydrated.

The Importance of Adequate Hydration

Proper hydration is vital for sustaining general health and well-being, as water is involved in several physiological processes within the body. Water acts as a fundamental component of biological fluids, including blood, lymph, and digestive juices, and plays a vital function in controlling body temperature, carrying nutrients and oxygen to cells, lubricating joints, and removing waste products through urine and sweat.

A variety of the key reasons hydration is so important is its impact on physical performance and cognitive function. Dehydration can affect physical performance, resulting in diminished endurance, strength, and coordination, as well as increased tiredness and perceived exertion during exercise. Inadequate hydration can also disrupt cognitive function, producing trouble concentrating, diminished awareness, and impaired decision-making skills.

Moreover, sufficient hydration is vital for preserving cardiovascular health and kidney function. Water helps regulate blood volume and pressure, ensuring appropriate circulation of oxygen and nutrients to cells throughout the body. Additionally, proper hydration improves kidney function by promoting the disposal of waste products and toxins through urine, decreasing the formation of kidney stones, and reducing the incidence of urinary tract infections.

Furthermore, water plays a key function in promoting gut health and nutritional absorption. Water helps soften and dissolve fiber, assisting in the digestion and absorption of nutrients from food. It also helps avoid constipation by keeping stools soft and promoting regular bowel motions. Adequate hydration is vital for maintaining good digestive function and preventing gastrointestinal disorders.

Overall, enough hydration is crucial for sustaining optimal health and well-being, supporting physical performance, cognitive function, cardiovascular health, kidney function, digestive health, and nutritional absorption.

Creative Ways to Stay Hydrated

While drinking simple water is the most obvious approach to staying hydrated, there are numerous inventive and entertaining ways to improve fluid intake throughout the day. Here are some inventive methods to remain hydrated:

Infused Water: Infusing water with fruits, vegetables, and herbs gives natural flavor and encourages hydration. Try adding slices of cucumber, lemon, lime, or strawberries to water for a refreshing and tasty beverage. Mint, basil, or ginger can also offer a burst of freshness and flavor to infused water.

Herbal Teas: Herbal teas are a hydrating alternative to plain water and offer a variety of flavors and health advantages. Brew herbal teas such as chamomile, peppermint, hibiscus, or ginger tea for a calming and hydrating beverage. Herbal teas are caffeine-free and can be sipped hot or cold.

Coconut Water: Coconut water is a natural and electrolyte-rich beverage that hydrates the body and restores lost electrolytes after exercise or physical activity. Enjoy coconut water as a pleasant and hydrating alternative to sugary sports drinks.

Smoothies and Juices: Smoothies and fresh juices produced from fruits and vegetables are refreshing and nutritious liquids that include necessary vitamins, minerals, and antioxidants. Blend fruits like watermelon, cucumber, or pineapple with water or coconut water for a hydrating and delicious smoothie.

Hydrating Foods: Many fruits and vegetables have significant water content and can contribute to hydration. Incorporate hydrating foods such as watermelon, cucumbers, strawberries, oranges, tomatoes, and celery into meals and snacks to enhance fluid consumption throughout the day.

Frozen Treats: Homemade popsicles prepared from pureed fruits or coconut water are a pleasant and hydrating treat, especially during hot weather. Freeze fruit purees or coconut water in popsicle molds for a delicious and hydrating dessert.

Soup and Broth: Enjoying soups and broths made from clear, vegetable-based stocks or bone broth is a hydrating method to absorb fluids while also supplying critical minerals and electrolytes. Choose low-sodium alternatives for a healthier decision.

Hydration Reminder Apps: Use smartphone apps designed to remind you to drink water consistently throughout the day. These applications can deliver notifications and reminders to help you remain on track with your hydration goals.

Hydration Stations: Create hydration stations in your home or workplace by placing pitchers or bottles of water flavored with fruits and herbs in convenient areas. Having readily available and visually appealing hydration options can encourage regular fluid intake.

Hydration Challenges: Participate in hydration challenges with friends, family, or coworkers to stay motivated and accountable for completing your hydration goals. Set explicit targets for daily water intake and track your progress together.

Hydration is energetic for maintaining overall wellness and supporting different biological processes, including physical performance, cognitive function, cardiovascular health, kidney function, digestive health, and nutrient absorption. While drinking plain water is the most straightforward way to stay hydrated, there are many creative and enjoyable ways to increase fluid intake throughout the day, such as infused water, herbal teas, coconut water, smoothies, hydrating foods, frozen treats, soup and broth, hydration reminder apps, hydration stations, and hydration challenges. By adopting these inventive ideas into your daily routine, you can keep hydrated and promote your overall health and well-being.

Chapter 10

Environmental Sustainability

In an era where the impact of human actions on the environment is becoming increasingly obvious, implementing methods that promote environmental sustainability is vital. This extends to our choices surrounding food – from what we eat to how we source and dispose of it. In this inquiry, we will delve into the necessity of making eco-friendly food choices and tactics for decreasing food waste, all with the goal of a more sustainable and ecologically conscious lifestyle.

Making Eco-Friendly Food Choices

Choosing Locally Sourced and Seasonal Produce: Opting for locally sourced and seasonal produce is a cornerstone of eco-friendly eating choices. Locally grown foods require less transportation, lowering the carbon footprint associated with their trip from farm to table. Seasonal produce also tends to be more abundant, increasing biodiversity and supporting local farmers.

Embracing Plant-Based Options: The environmental impact of animal production, particularly red meat, is well-documented. Livestock production contributes greatly to deforestation, greenhouse gas emissions, and water pollution. Choosing plant-based options or introducing more plant-based meals into your diet will dramatically minimize your ecological impact. Plant-based proteins including beans, tofu, and tempeh offer sustainable alternatives.

Prioritizing Sustainable Seafood: If seafood is part of your diet, opting for sustainable choices can contribute to the health of oceans and marine ecosystems. Certain fishing tactics can lead to overfishing and harm to non-target species. Look for certifications such as the Marine Stewardship Council (MSC) or Best Aquaculture Practices (BAP) when purchasing seafood to guarantee it comes from properly managed sources.

Reducing Single-Use Plastics: The excessive use of single-use plastics in packaging adds to pollution and poses a threat to marine life. Choose products with minimum or eco-friendly packaging, and consider taking your reusable bags, containers, and utensils while shopping or dining out. Reducing reliance on single-use plastics is a tiny but impactful step towards a more sustainable food system.

Supporting Local Farmers and Sustainable Practices: Building a connection with local farmers and supporting sustainable farming practices is vital to eco-friendly food choices. Familiarize yourself with the practices of local farmers and buy products from those implementing environmentally responsible methods such as organic farming, agroforestry, or regenerative agriculture. Supporting such approaches helps a shift towards more sustainable food production.

Reducing Food Waste

Understanding Expiry Dates and Proper Storage: A key contributor to food wastage is the misunderstanding of expiration dates. Many individuals reject food early based on these dates, adding to wasteful waste. Understanding the distinction between "sell by," "use by," and "best before" dates can prevent premature disposal. Proper storage methods, such as refrigerating perishables promptly, also play a key role in avoiding food wastage.

Meal Planning and Batch Cooking: Planning meals and batch cooking can be useful ways to decrease food waste. By knowing what ingredients, you have and preparing meals accordingly, you can purchase only what you need, lowering the possibility of wasted things rotting. Batch cooking allows you to produce greater quantities and store leftovers for future meals, lowering the odds of items going to waste.

Creative Use of Leftovers: Transforming leftovers into fresh and intriguing dishes is a creative method to reduce food waste. Repurposing cooked veggies into soups, salads, or stir-fries, and using surplus grains or proteins in new recipes can provide variety to your meals while saving food from being thrown. Embracing culinary innovation is not only pleasurable but also adds to a more sustainable kitchen.

Composting: Composting is a valuable strategy for handling food waste responsibly. Fruit and vegetable scraps, coffee grounds, eggshells, and other compostable materials can be transformed into nutrient-rich compost for gardens or plants. Setting up a composting system at home or participating in community composting programs diverts organic waste from landfills, where it would otherwise emit harmful methane gas.

Donating Surplus Food: In communities where food insecurity is an issue, donating surplus food to local charities, shelters, or food banks is a significant method to battle both food waste and hunger. Many charities take non-perishable products as well as fresh produce and prepared meals. This method not only minimizes waste but also aids in addressing socioeconomic challenges related to food accessibility.

Educating and Raising Awareness: Education is a powerful instrument in the fight against food waste. Raising awareness about the environmental impact of wasting food and providing practical tips for decreasing waste can empower individuals and communities to make better-informed decisions. Sharing knowledge about correct storage, portion management, and inventive cooking techniques can contribute to a greater culture of waste reduction.

Technology Solutions: In the digital era, technology can be harnessed to combat food waste. Apps and platforms that connect consumers with extra food from local retailers or restaurants at discounted prices might help reroute edible products that might otherwise go to waste. Similarly, applications that provide recipe suggestions based on available ingredients might urge users to use what they have on hand, eliminating wasteful expenditures and waste.

Environmental sustainability in the realm of food choices is a multidimensional activity that entails thoughtful decision-making at numerous stages of the food supply chain. From picking eco-friendly products and lowering reliance on single-use plastics to practicing ethical food consumption habits and eliminating waste, individuals can play a crucial role in building a more sustainable food system. By making educated decisions and adopting thoughtful behaviors, we contribute to a healthier planet and a more sustainable future for generations to come.

Chapter 11

Social and Cultural Influences on Eating

Eating is not merely a biological necessity but a social and cultural practice firmly woven into human existence. The way we eat is impacted by a multiplicity of circumstances, including social settings, cultural standards, and traditions. In this discussion, we will look into the subtle interplay between social and cultural influences that shape our eating patterns and cover tactics for navigating social settings, dining out, and healthily honoring food traditions.

Understanding Social and Cultural Influences on Eating

Social Dynamics and Food Choices: Humans are naturally social beings, and our eating habits are deeply influenced by the dynamics of social relationships. From family dinners to shared lunches at work, the presence of people typically determines what, when, and how much we eat. Social interactions can either support healthy eating habits through positive impacts or lead to poor choices due to peer pressure or cultural standards.

Cultural Traditions and Food Rituals: Cultural traditions and food rituals play a key role in molding our connection with food. From the significance of holiday feasts to the comfort of traditional recipes passed down through generations, cultural practices contribute to the way we view and experience food. These traditions frequently contain great emotional and community importance, generating a sense of identity and belonging.

Socialization of Eating Habits: From an early age, individuals are socialized into distinct eating habits by observing and mimicking the behaviors of those around them. Family meals, in particular, serve as a significant backdrop for the transfer of cultural norms and dietary behaviors. The foods we grow up consuming and the rituals surrounding meals become engrained in our personalities.

impacts of Media and Advertising: The ubiquitous effect of media and advertising further helps to shape our eating habits. Food ads, celebrity endorsements, and cultural portrayals of idealized body models can dramatically alter perceptions of what is deemed desirable or acceptable in terms of food consumption. These effects can, in turn, affect eating preferences and habits.

Navigating Social Settings and Dining Out

Balancing Social Enjoyment and Health Goals: Social situations generally focus on shared meals, whether at family gatherings, celebrations, or informal outings with friends. Navigating these scenarios while keeping health objectives can be tough. It's crucial to achieve a balance between enjoying the social part of eating and making mindful, health-conscious choices. Communicating your food choices or constraints might help develop understanding among peers.

Making Informed Restaurant Choices: Dining out brings unique obstacles, as restaurant menus may not necessarily correspond with individual health goals. However, making informed decisions at restaurants is doable. Look for menu options that highlight fresh, whole ingredients, and consider asking for alterations to fit your dietary needs. Many restaurants now provide healthier choices and are sensitive to unique demands.

Portion Control in Social Settings: Social settings typically come with larger amounts and the temptation to overindulge. Implementing tactics such as sharing dishes, choosing for smaller servings, or carrying leftovers can help manage portion sizes. Additionally, listening to your body's hunger and fullness cues rather than succumbing to external influences might help to a healthy relationship with food in social circumstances.

Choosing Mindful Eating Practices: Practicing mindful eating in social contexts requires being completely present throughout meals, relishing each bite, and paying attention to hunger and satiety cues.

This method not only enhances the dining experience but also creates a more conscientious relationship with food. By slowing down and enjoying the flavors, individuals can make more purposeful choices about what and how much they consume.

Preparing for Social situations: Preparing for social situations by planning helps empower individuals to make better choices.

Eating a short, nutrient-dense snack before attending an event can alleviate excessive appetite and prevent overeating. Additionally, bringing a meal to share guarantees that there are healthy options available and helps the social component of the gathering.

Celebrating Food Traditions in a Healthy Way

Adapting Traditional Recipes: Celebrating dietary traditions does not have to be at odds with health aims. Adapting traditional recipes by using healthier ingredients or altering cooking methods can keep the essence of the tradition while improving nutritional value. For example, switching whole grains for refined grains or eliminating added sugars might boost the health profile of a dish.

Integrating different Flavors: Exploring different flavors and cuisines offers for a diversified and enjoyable culinary experience while promoting health-conscious choices. Integrating components from diverse cultures might introduce new and delectable options that correspond with dietary preferences. This method broadens the culinary pallet and encourages a more open and adventurous approach to food.

Fostering a Positive Food Environment: Creating a positive food environment during celebrations entails more than just the sort of dishes provided. It also incorporates the atmosphere, the people present, and the overall attitude towards eating. Cultivating an environment that stresses enjoyment, thankfulness, and shared experiences rather than focusing exclusively on the meal itself adds to a healthier and more holistic celebration.

Encouraging Family and Community Involvement: Food traditions frequently entail the participation of family and community members. Engaging in the cooking of traditional cuisine as a collaborative activity develops a sense of connection and shared responsibility. This collaborative endeavor not only develops ties but also allows for the exchange of culinary expertise and skills across generations.

Balancing Indulgence and Moderation: Celebrations typically come with sumptuous foods and exceptional dishes. Balancing excess with moderation is crucial to maintaining a healthy approach to food during festive events. Enjoying classic sweets or fatty dishes in moderation and balancing them with nutrient-dense options ensures a delightful experience without compromising health goals.

Social and cultural impacts on eating are profoundly ingrained in human behavior, affecting our relationship with food from an early age. Navigating social environments, dining

Chapter 12

Discover how food can heal your body and improve your health

In addition to being a source of sustenance, food has long been recognized as an effective means for promoting health and healing within the body. This recognition dates back a long time. Because the foods we consume have a considerable influence on defining our overall well-being, the proverb "you are what you eat" carries a great deal of truth. In recent years, there has been a growing awareness of the therapeutic potential of food. Research has shown the tremendous impact that dietary choices have on numerous areas of health, and this knowledge has led to an increase in scientific understanding. There is no denying the fact that food has the ability to heal, as evidenced by the fact that it can lower the risk of developing chronic diseases, boost immune function, and improve mental well-being.

For optimal health, nutrient-dense foods provide the body with the fuel it needs.

The concept of having a diet that is rich in nutrients and supplies the body with the critical vitamins, minerals, antioxidants, and other bioactive compounds that are required for optimal functioning is at the heart of the practice of using food as medicine. The foundation of a healthy diet is comprised of foods that are abundant in nutrients, such as fruits, vegetables, whole grains, lean proteins, and healthy fats. These meals are loaded with vitamins and minerals that support a variety of biological activities, including the metabolism of energy, the function of the immune system, and the healing of injured cells.

Fruits and Vegetables: Fruits and vegetables are nutritional powerhouses, packed to the brim with vitamins, minerals, and phytonutrients that are beneficial to one's general health. The consumption of a diet that includes a wide variety of colorful fruits and vegetables leads to the consumption of a wide variety of nutrients that are beneficial to one's health and vigor. From vitamin C-rich citrus fruits to beta-carotene-packed leafy greens, each plant-based meal offers unique health benefits.

Whole Grains: Whole grains, such as oats, quinoa, brown rice, and whole wheat, are rich in fiber, vitamins, and minerals. Unlike processed grains, which have been stripped of their nutrient-rich bran and germ layers, whole grains preserve their nutritional integrity. Consuming whole grains improves digestive health, maintains blood sugar levels, and reduces the risk of chronic diseases like heart disease and type 2 diabetes.

Lean Proteins: Protein is needed for creating and repairing tissues, supporting immunological function, and maintaining muscular mass. Lean protein sources, such as poultry, fish, tofu, lentils, and nuts, provide high-quality protein without excessive saturated fat or cholesterol. Including a range of lean proteins in the diet ensures optimal consumption of key amino acids necessary for overall health.

Healthy Fats: Healthy fats, including monounsaturated and polyunsaturated fats found in foods like avocados, olive oil, almonds, and fatty fish, play a critical role in maintaining heart health, brain function, and hormone synthesis. Incorporating these beneficial fats into the diet in moderation helps maintain appropriate cholesterol levels and minimizes the risk of cardiovascular disease.

The Healing Power of Phytonutrients

In addition to important vitamins and minerals, many plant-based diets contain phytonutrients, bioactive molecules with significant antioxidant and anti-inflammatory activities. Phytonutrients, also known as phytochemicals, give fruits, vegetables, herbs, and spices their brilliant colors, tastes, and fragrances. These substances have been linked to a plethora of health advantages, including lower inflammation, increased immunological function, and enhanced detoxification mechanisms within the body.

Flavonoids: Flavonoids are a varied group of phytonutrients found in fruits, vegetables, tea, and cocoa. They are recognized for their antioxidant and anti-inflammatory qualities and have been connected with a reduced risk of chronic diseases like heart disease, cancer, and neurological disorders. Foods rich in flavonoids include berries, citrus fruits, apples, onions, and dark leafy greens.

Carotenoids: Carotenoids are pigments found in fruits and vegetables that give them their brilliant colors. These chemicals, including beta-carotene, lutein, and lycopene, have antioxidant characteristics and have a role in supporting eye health, immunological function, and skin health. Carotenoid-rich foods include carrots, sweet potatoes, tomatoes, spinach, and bell peppers.

Polyphenols: Polyphenols are a broad set of phytonutrients found in foods including tea, coffee, berries, nuts, and dark chocolate. These chemicals contain antioxidant and anti-inflammatory characteristics and have been linked to a reduced risk of chronic diseases such as heart disease, cancer, and neurological disorders. Polyphenols may also enhance gut health by increasing the growth of healthy gut flora.

Sulfur Compounds: Sulfur compounds present in foods like garlic, onions, cruciferous vegetables (such as broccoli, cabbage, and Brussels sprouts), and allium vegetables (such as leeks and shallots) have been researched for their possible health advantages. These chemicals have antioxidant and anti-inflammatory properties and may help detoxification processes within the body. Additionally, sulfur compounds present in garlic have been linked to cardiovascular health advantages.

Supporting Immune Function and Fighting Inflammation

A well-balanced diet rich in minerals and phytonutrients has a critical role in boosting immune function and lowering inflammation within the body. The immune system needs a range of vitamins and minerals, including vitamins A, C, D, E, zinc, and selenium, to function efficiently. These nutrients help control immune responses, increase the creation of immune cells, and boost the body's fight against infections and disorders.

Vitamin C: Vitamin C is a strong antioxidant that supports immune function by boosting the development of white blood cells, which help fight off infections. Food are rich in vitamin C contain citrus fruits (such as oranges, lemons, and grapefruits).

Chapter 13

Learn how eating fruits can benefit your health

Fruits are nature's delectable and nutrient-packed gifts, giving a myriad of health advantages that contribute to overall well-being. From colorful berries to delicious citrus fruits, each kind delivers its distinct combination of vitamins, minerals, antioxidants, and fiber. In this study, we will delve into the broad array of health advantages connected with including fruits in your diet, highlighting how these beautiful beauties can increase your health and vitality.

Nutrient Powerhouses

Fruits are nutritious powerhouses, delivering critical vitamins and minerals that are required for many biological activities. They are rich in vitamin C, an antioxidant that helps immunological function, collagen formation, and wound healing. Additionally, fruits such as bananas and avocados are excellent providers of potassium, which helps control blood pressure and maintain appropriate muscle and nerve function.

Antioxidant Protection

Many fruits are rich in antioxidants, chemicals that help neutralize damaging free radicals and protect the body against oxidative stress and inflammation. Berries, in particular, are recognized for their high antioxidant content, with kinds like blueberries, strawberries, and raspberries having exceptional levels of anthocyanins, flavonoids, and other phytochemicals that improve cellular health and reduce the risk of chronic diseases.

Heart Health Support

Regular eating of fruits has been connected with a lower risk of heart disease and stroke. Fruits including apples, grapes, and citrus fruits include soluble fiber, which helps decrease cholesterol levels and promote heart health. Furthermore, potassium-rich foods like bananas and oranges assist regulate blood pressure, reducing the risk of hypertension and cardiovascular problems.

Weight Management

Incorporating fruits into your diet might be useful for weight management and maintenance. Fruits are naturally low in calories and fat while being high in fiber, which promotes satiety and helps regulate hunger. By picking fruits as snacks or incorporating them into meals, you can fulfill demands for sweetness while keeping calorie intake in line, making it simpler to maintain a healthy weight.

Digestive Health

Fruits are high in dietary fiber, which plays a critical role in promoting digestive health. Fiber adds weight to stool, supporting regular bowel motions and reducing constipation. Additionally, many fruits, such as papayas and pineapples, include enzymes like papain and bromelain, which aid in digestion by breaking down proteins and improving nutrient absorption.

Blood Sugar Regulation

Contrary to prevalent assumptions, most fruits have a low glycemic index (GI), meaning they cause a gradual and consistent increase in blood sugar levels rather than a fast spike. This makes fruits acceptable for those with diabetes or those attempting to manage blood sugar levels. Choosing whole fruits over fruit juices or dried fruits will further assist manage blood sugar levels and minimize insulin spikes.

Cancer Prevention

The antioxidants and phytochemicals present in fruits have been linked to a lower risk of some forms of cancer. For example, citrus fruits include chemicals like limonoids and flavonoids, which have shown anti-cancer benefits in laboratory experiments. Similarly, berries include anthocyanins and ellagic acid, which display anti-inflammatory and anti-carcinogenic properties.

Skin Health and Aging

The vitamins and antioxidants included in fruits contribute to skin health and combat indications of aging. Vitamin C, in particular, is necessary for collagen formation, which helps preserve skin suppleness and firmness. Additionally, antioxidants like vitamin E and beta-carotene protect the skin from oxidative damage caused by UV radiation and environmental contaminants, helping to preserve a youthful complexion.

Boosting Immune Function

Fruits are rich in immune-boosting elements including vitamin C, vitamin A, and zinc, which assist the body's defensive mechanisms against infections and illnesses. Vitamin C, in particular, plays a critical role in improving immune function by increasing the formation of white blood cells and antibodies. Regular eating of fruits can boost the immune system and lower the risk of common colds and infections.

Brain Health and Cognitive Function

The antioxidants and phytochemicals included in fruits have been related to increased brain health and cognitive performance. Studies have revealed that certain fruits, such as berries and grapes, contain chemicals that may help protect against age-related cognitive decline and neurodegenerative disorders like Alzheimer's and Parkinson's. Additionally, fruits high in flavonoids and polyphenols have been related to better memory, attention, and learning capacities.

Improving Hydration

Many fruits have significant water content, making them good hydrating snacks, especially during hot weather or after strenuous exertion. Water-rich fruits like watermelon, strawberries, and cucumbers not only assist restore fluids but also give critical electrolytes like potassium and magnesium, which are lost through sweat.

Including Fruits into Your Diet

Incorporating a variety of fruits into your regular diet is straightforward and fun. Fresh fruits can be enjoyed on their own as snacks or mixed with other foods like salads, smoothies, oats, yogurt parfaits, and desserts. Frozen fruits are easy options for adding to smoothies or baking into muffins and bread. Canned fruits, ideally those packed in water or natural juice without added sugars, are convenient cupboard staples for quick and easy meal additions.

Fruits are not only delicious but also highly useful for health, giving a wide range of nutrients, antioxidants, and health-promoting substances. By including a variety of fruits into your diet regularly, you may support your general health and well-being, from boosting immunity and protecting against chronic diseases to improving skin health and supporting cognitive function. So next time you go for a snack, consider reaching for a piece of fruit and savor the various benefits it has to offer.

Conclusion

As we draw the curtain on this journey into understanding good eating habits and sustainable lifestyle choices, it is natural to reflect on the depth of insights obtained and the transformational potential that lies within adopting a lifetime of nutrient-rich eating. your last chapter acts as a compass, pointing you towards not just the completion of your research but the commencement of a sustainable and healthy lifestyle that vibrates with vitality and well-being.

Reflecting on Your Journey

Reflection is a great tool for human growth and knowledge. Throughout this study, you've traversed through the complicated terrain of nutrition, delving into the science of nutrients, analyzing the advantages of numerous foods, and understanding the significant impact of lifestyle choices on overall health. Take a minute to reflect on the knowledge obtained, the behaviors you've reassessed, and the mindfulness cultivated around your relationship with food and the environment.

Consider the dietary shifts you've made, the mindful eating practices you've embraced, and the understanding generated around the interconnectivity of food, health, and the world around you. Reflect on the challenges faced and the achievements experienced. Acknowledge the strides gained towards developing a healthier, more sustainable living. This introspection is not just about what you've learned but how this information has converted into beneficial behaviors in your daily life.

Embracing a Lifetime of Nutrient-Rich Eating

The concept of nutrient-rich eating goes beyond a mere dietary choice; it encompasses a philosophy that views food as a source of nourishment, healing, and resilience. As you move forward, consider embracing a lifetime commitment to nutrient-rich eating, a journey that promotes full, authentic foods brimming with critical vitamins, minerals, antioxidants, and fiber.

Creating a Balanced Plate: Building a balanced plate includes adding a variety of nutrient-dense foods in the proper quantities. Focus on colorful fruits and vegetables, entire grains, lean proteins, and healthy fats. By broadening your meal, you ensure a broad spectrum of nutrients required for overall health and well-being.

Portion Control and Food Groups: Practicing portion control is a sustainable technique for reducing calorie intake and promoting mindful eating. Recognize the value of several dietary groups, realizing that each supply specific nutrients. Strive for a harmonious balance that recognizes both your nutritional demands and enjoyment of food.

The Power of Colorful Eating: The brilliance of colors in fruits and vegetables suggests a vast array of nutrients. Embrace the power of a colorful diet, where each hue signifies a distinct collection of health-promoting substances. From the antioxidants in berries to the beta-carotene in carrots, let your meal be a canvas of nutrients.

Embracing a Sustainable Lifestyle

Sustainability extends beyond individual health to the well-being of the world. Embracing a sustainable lifestyle entails deliberate choices that evaluate the environmental impact of our actions. As you go on this journey, bear these ideas in mind.

Mindful Eating Techniques: Extend the practice of awareness beyond the act of eating itself. Cultivate mindfulness in all stages of your food journey – from shopping for groceries to cooking meals. Choose locally produced, seasonal vegetables when possible, decreasing the carbon footprint associated with food transportation.

Environmental Sustainability: Make eco-friendly food choices by supporting sustainable farming techniques. Opt for organic produce to avoid exposure to chemicals and contribute to soil health. Consider limiting meat intake or choosing ethically sourced and responsibly grown foods to solve environmental concerns linked with large-scale animal husbandry.

Reducing Food Waste: Combatting food waste is an important element of sustainability. Plan meals wisely, utilize leftovers imaginatively, and be mindful of expiration dates. Composting organic waste adds to soil fertility, closing the loop in the food cycle and lowering the strain on landfills.

A Vision for the Future

As you embrace a lifetime of nutrient-rich nutrition and sustainable lifestyle choices, visualize the ripple effect it can have on your health and the world. Imagine a future where individuals make conscious choices, not only for personal well-being but for the larger good. Visualize communities thriving on the concepts of nutrition, sustainability, and mindful living.

In this future, nutrient-rich foods are accessible to anyone, independent of socioeconomic factors. Sustainable practices are interwoven into mainstream living, impacting legislation, corporations, and consumer behaviors. The influence of our collective choices reverberates in the health of individuals and the health of the planet, creating a harmonious coexistence.

The Continuing Journey

This conclusion is not an endpoint but a juncture in your ongoing journey toward well-being and sustainability. The knowledge you've received and the habits you've accepted are foundational stones for a lifetime of positive decisions. Carry this insight forward, sharing it with others and encouraging a ripple effect of health-conscious living.

In the continuum of your journey, let curiosity be your guide, discovery be your companion, and well-being be your destination. Each meal is an opportunity, each choice a step towards a healthier you and a healthy world. As you relish the pleasures of nutrient-rich meals and adopt sustainable behaviors, remember that this trip is not just about the destination but the delight found in every mindful and intentional step along the way.